MEDITERRANEAN DIET FOR HEART HEALTH AND WEIGHT LOSS

MY 24 WEEKS RESEARCH AND FINDINGS WITH 5 OVERWEIGHT PEOPLE ON MEDITERRANEAN DIET

BY

JENNIFER ROBSON

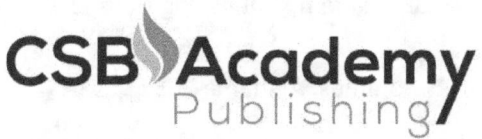

Copyrights

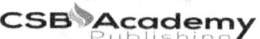

CSB Academy Publishing Company.
P. O. Box 966
Semmes, Alabama 36575, USA

Cover Designed

By

David Miller

First Edition

Table of Contents

Introduction

"To keep the body in good health is a duty... otherwise, we shall not be able to keep our mind strong and clear" -Buddha

This is the time we should be most conscious of our diet, but most of us aren't at all. The dietary lifestyle of Americans hasn't changed for the better but for the worst. Escalating reliance on ready-to-cook and fast foods have given rise to the obesity culture, which is detrimental to health. In the US, the leading cause of death among men and women is heart disease, causing about 610,000 deaths each year; to put the stats into better perspective, this means 1 in 4 deaths.

However, apart from the diet, the problem also lies in how actively we are leading our lives. Doing our daily chores and activities doesn't constitute a healthy and active lifestyle, but we are continuing with it. What should our diet ideally constitute of? How can we lead an active life? These are all questions which led me to explore the different diets out there to determine **the best way to live a healthy life and lose weight effectively.**

This book is part of a three-book diet series where I take a research-based approach and explore the ins and outs of three popular diets. In my first book, I have talked about the ketogenic diet and my research, which validates that its one of the best low car diets to lose weight provided that you follow it carefully and with devotion.

In this book, I discuss the Mediterranean diet, its benefits, and how it can help steer you towards a healthy lifestyle. Being a freelance researcher gives me many avenues to conduct research and I've been associated with a number of organizations over time to conduct different kinds of research for them. This research on the Mediterranean diet was conducted with the purpose of finding the truth about the diet, its effectiveness, and ideas to implement it in daily life with relative ease. At the time this research was conducted, I could not publish it due to my contract with the company, but now that the period has elapsed, I am free to share my results with you.

What I found out about this particular diet is astounding to say the least. Not only did the participants of my research lose considerable weight but started to feel great about themselves too. Their lives changed for the better, and they are thankful they took the first step towards a healthy lifestyle. When you make positive diet changes in your life, it doesn't only affect your body, but your overall wellness allowing you to lead a fulfilled life.

I can't wait to share my research experience on the Mediterranean diet with you, and I hope you benefit from it as much as my research participants did.

Good Luck!

A big Thank you for buying my book, I appreciate it. I am not a writer but wanted to share some of my knowledge with everyone.

If you like my work, please give me a review on Amazon.

Thanks again!

Chapter 1: What Is the Mediterranean Diet

The Mediterranean diet has carved its place as one of the healthiest diets out there, which helps develop a positive lifestyle. Many research studies have been conducted on this dietary lifestyle of the people of the Mediterranean Sea and surrounding areas validating that it helps develop and maintain healthy eating habits effectively. The Mediterranean diet is about not only the foods you include in your daily diet but also the overall lifestyle changes that you make. It includes activities, meals, foods and even the intake of wine in moderation to develop a long lasting diet plan that is healthy.

In essence, the Mediterranean diet includes fruits, vegetables, legumes and grains as well as fish and chicken in moderate quantity. Unsaturated fat and red meat is allowed in little amounts, and most of the fat is derived from olive and nuts. Red wine in moderation can also help provide health benefits.

In 2013, a study found that people who followed the Mediterranean diet had a 30 percent lower risk of heart disease and stroke. It is essentially the diet, which the people in Italy, Greece, Spain, and France follow for the most part, but researchers have concluded that it's not just the diet that is their secret to a healthy life but their overall lifestyle, which includes exercise and living a fit life.

The Harvard school of public health, Oldways, and the European office of the World Health Organization (WHO) introduced the classic Mediterranean diet in 1993. They also presented a Mediterranean diet pyramid graphic which serves as the gold standard or guide to the eating patterns that should be developed for lifelong good health. It is widely researched and used by consumers as well as health professionals to develop healthier eating habits. The plan is based on the dietary traditions of Greece, southern Italy, and Crete at a time when the chronic disease rates in their populations were the lowest and the adult life expectancy rates were among the highest, in the world given that medical services were limited at that time.

The key to the success of the Mediterranean diet

It is clear that the success of the Mediterranean diet is attributed to its resistance to today's modernized foods, which have become an essential part of our new diets over the past 50 years or so. These modernized foods have introduced us to eating less healthier and fresh vegetables and fruits, more meat, and processed foods which have collectively contributed to the increased dilemma of obesity, diabetes, heart disease and other chronic diseases.

The diet of the people of the Mediterranean countries was considered a "poor" diet as they only relied on fruits, nuts, grains, vegetables, olive oil, fish, and small amounts of dairy and red wine to make up their diet. This contributed to their lifelong good health, being regarded today as healthy eating, which everyone should be adopting.

The Food Pyramid

There may be some variations in the eating and diet patterns of Mediterranean diet of different regions but with little or no differences, all sticking to some basic rules, which were also defined in the food pyramid. More or less the aim of the diet is to foster healthy eating habits derived from the natural nutrition source of food, exercise and celebrate the happiness of mealtime. It is noted that when families sit together to have food it creates feelings of goodwill and meals should be shared with others to double their effect. The basics of the food pyramid include:

- Eating plant-based foods in abundances such as potatoes, vegetables, fruits, beans, nuts, seeds, and grains.

- Replacing other fats and oils such as butter and margarine and making olive oil the principal source of fat.
- Eliminating and minimizing processed foods from the diet and switching to locally grown foods due to their micronutrient content that benefits health as well as the presence of antioxidants.
- Keeping the total fats between 25 percent to 35 percent of caloric intake with saturated fats limited to 8 percent of caloric intake
- Intake of fish and poultry only two days a week in moderate amounts
- Cheese and yogurt can be consumed in moderation on daily basis
- Include red meat in diet only a few times in a month limited to an intake of 12-16 ounces each month. If possible, opt for lean meat.

What Led To Its Discovery?

The Mediterranean diet was discovered by a physiologist by the name of Ancel Keys who did not regard heart diseases as a necessary part of the aging process in the 1950s. He laid the foundation for this diet which today is known as the Mediterranean diet and proved by living to a hundred years old that it was possible to defeat ill health and heart diseases if only one would resort to eating healthy.

The first large-scale study that took place included 22,000 healthy adults in Greece, and it was found that eating foods prescribed on the Mediterranean diet helped reduce death due to heart disease and cancer significantly. Before 2003, no such studies that validated findings through concrete data had been carried out although there were a number of studies that took place. In this study, the participants were followed over time, and their diets were evaluated for a year prior to data collection by Dr. Trichopoulou and his colleagues. Nine dietary components were looked at in the study and for each dietary category a value of 0 or 1 was assigned. 1 was assigned when a participant ate a diet higher in one of the nine dietary components. A value of 0 indicated a western diet while the value 1 was indicative of a perfect Mediterranean style diet. It was found that even small dietary changes had a big impact, and those had better scores indeed lived longer. According to the study a 2 point improvement on the scale from 2 to 5 translated into a 25% reduction in death related to heart disease. This indicates that adding healthy vegetables and legumes to the diet can significantly improve health.

Research Studies on the Mediterranean Diet

If you are looking for more validation about the Mediterranean diet as a way to live a healthy life and decrease the risks of heart disease then you can feel safe in the knowledge that there are indeed many studies conducted on this particular diet and all of them lead to only one conclusion: you can decrease your risk of heart disease by following the Mediterranean diet.

A study published in 2013, the PREDIMED study found that following this diet led to a significant decrease in cardiovascular risk. It studied a total number of 7447 individuals suffering from cardiovascular disease and were randomly assigned to three different Mediterranean diet patterns which were:

- Low-fat control group
- Mediterranean diet with nuts
- Mediterranean diet with extra virgin olive oil

The study went on for five years without limiting participants' caloric intake or increasing their physical activity, and a variety of results were concluded with this research which looked at different aspects and implications of the diet. In one paper published in The New England Journal of Medicine they looked at the risk of heart attack, stroke and death as a result of cardiovascular reasons and found that it was decreased by 330% in people on the Mediterranean + olive oil group and 28% in the Mediterranean + nuts group. Those people who suffered from high blood pressure, obesity and lipid problems were seen to respond the best to this type of diet.

Another research published in the JAMA Internal Medicine looked at a sample of 372 individuals from the study after three months to evaluate changes in oxidative stress markers like oxidized LDL. Decreased levels of oxidized LDL were found in people part of the Mediterranean diet groups.

The diet groups also showed some promising results for diabetes. In a study published in Diabetes Care, 418 participants who were non-diabetic were assessed for four years to evaluate their risk of developing type 2 diabetes. It was found that the 11 percent of the people on Mediterranean diet became diabetic in the four years compared to 17.9% in the low-fat control group. Furthermore, the participants of the Mediterranean diet group had a 52% reduced risk of developing type 2 diabetes.

In a nutshell, it can be concluded that following a Mediterranean diet leads to lower risk of heart disease, blood sugar, diabetes, cardiovascular diseases, heart stroke and obesity. It is one of the most recommended diets by doctors for patients who suffer from high cholesterol and heart conditions. Consumption of nuts and olive oil are the prime reasons which help reduce these risks on the Mediterranean diet.

Chapter2: Basic Rules of the Mediterranean Diet

The Mediterranean diet is based on the notion that food should be enjoyed. It sees cooking, eating and cleaning the table as a function that should be performed together. Everyone should sit together to have their food thus emphasizing the importance of sharing and caring while having food. The American lifestyle and diet pattern has given way to secluded eating due to the busy life schedule of parents and children. Everyone eats food when and as they feel like it and it is often not together. This diet emphasizes that you sit together with friends and family to enjoy your food.

It includes being involved in grocery purchasing, deciding the menu, cooking the food, finding out new healthy recipes to try and sitting together to enjoy the final meal. These things contribute to physical and mental health when family or friends unite over food to discuss their day's events, share their problems, and find mutual solutions and just talk. It helps people feel lighter, and there are fewer feelings that stay bottled up inside.

Some basic things to keep in mind when following the Mediterranean diet include:

8 Key Points to Consider

Include plant based foods

The majority of the foods that are part of the Mediterranean diet are those which come from plants. For example, you can include nuts, seeds, whole grains, fruits and vegetables, herbs, spices, olive oil. Any season's fruits and vegetables are also strongly encouraged to be included in the diet.

Season with herbs and spices

The Mediterranean diet foods and dishes can be seasoned with herbs and spices to create a strong flavor that enhances taste and generates food interest. When adding herbs and spices to season food, it will help cut down any added salt, sugar and fat that you are used to adding while cooking the foods. To add flavor to dishes, citrus juice can also be used.

Use olive oil for cooking

All dishes and cuisines cooked on this diet should be cooked using olive oil as the staple fat. Limit or eliminate your use of margarine, butter and other solid fats in cooking as these are high in saturated and trans fats that damage arteries and contributes to increase in cholesterol levels.

On the other hand, using olive oil is beneficial as it contains monounsaturated fats which are a type of healthy fat that helps keep the cholesterol levels low.

Include whole grains, nuts, beans, and legumes

Apart from an abundant and healthy source of vegetables and fruits other foods that should be part of your daily diet should include beans and whole grains as they are a healthy form of carbohydrate. Nuts contain healthy unsaturated fats and are very favorable on the Mediterranean diet plan.

Include lean protein and fish twice a week

To add a bit of variety to the diet while ensuring that it does not break the dietary rules as well lean protein and fish is allowed twice a week. Fish is a source of animal protein, and some forms contain omega 3 fatty acids which are good for brain and heart health. You can include herring, sardines, mackerel, halibut, albacore tuna, salmon, and trout two days in a week in your diet plan.

Few times in a week you can also include eggs, cheese, chicken and low-fat dairy eggs but remember to include hem in small portions. Traditional Mediterranean eating does not include or encourage the consumption of red meat but if you must and/ or you are following the not so traditional Mediterranean diet, you must still limit your intake of red meat and poultry to 3 ounces or less in a week.

Limit intake of high sugar foods and sweets

Deserts and fruit inspired sweet dishes can be enjoyed on the Mediterranean diet but in a limited quantity. You can indulge in a dessert once in a while, but that should be in manageable size portion only to satisfy your sweet tooth

Include moderate amount of alcohol (optional)

Moderate amount of alcohol consumption is part of the Mediterranean diet but it is optional and depends on the person likeness whether they would want to make wine a part of their diet or not. It is very important to include a good amount of water but if you include alcohol as well then women should not drink more than 1 drink in a day and men should not have more than 2 drinks in a day as part of their diet plan. One drink means a 5-ounce portion that equals just a little above half a cup.

Stay active

A big contribution to the success of the Mediterranean diet is staying active which is also seen as part of the lifestyle and culture of the traditional Mediterranean people. As part of your daily routine, you should include walking and other kinds of physical activity to remain active such as running, jogging or exercise as your age allows you to do.

 Following this diet isn't only about the foods you intake but overall how healthy your lifestyle is. Do you drive to even the nearest store? Do you sit for long hours at your workstation? These are also signs of an unhealthy lifestyle and which you should be aiming to change. Stay active in all the work that you do remember to stretch in between periods of long sitting or standing to give your muscles a break. If possible and suitable include going to the gym in your schedule. These are all the things that you can even do with your peers, friends or family to keep yourself motivated and focused.

The Mediterranean diet is a good choice of adoption for people with diabetes, those who want to lose weight or even if you are setting out to eat healthier. It involves including well balanced and controlled foods and portion sizes to you diet. In a nutshell you must remember to:

- Fill at least ½ your plate with non-starchy vegetables.
- Focus on adding more fruits and vegetables to your diet.
- Include whole grains and beans and other forms of healthy carbohydrates
- Choose healthy unsaturated fats
- Include fish and lean proteins twice a week
- Limit sweet desserts and intake of sugars
- Add physical activity to the routine.

Myths Associated With the Diet

Like any other diet, the Mediterranean diet is also surrounded by a range of different myths that can make the diet difficult for anyone to follow. However, with the benefits that this diet extends, it's hard to not shed light on these myths and help you understand that it is an easy diet to follow which helps lead a healthy life as well. Consider these common myths you will often come across when planning to follow the Mediterranean diet and decide for yourself whether its benefits outweighs it drawbacks and there is any truth in these myths:

It Is Expensive

The first thing you will often come across when following the Mediterranean diet is that it's expensive. The fact is that all meals prepared on this diet are prepared from lentils or beans which are the source of protein. Sticking to plant-based foods does not make it expensive but the contrary when compared to the meat, cheese, and processed foods based diet.

Eating Large Bowls of Pasta and Bread Is the Way to Follow the Mediterranean Diet

Eating a big bowl of pasta isn't the Mediterranean diet but, in fact, the American way of consuming pasta. Pasta is usually a side dish on the plate with a ½ to 1 cup of serving. Other components on the plate should include vegetables, salads, and a slice of bread and a small portion of meat.

It's only about the Food

Food makes up a large part of the diet, but it's not all about that. The way you consume food and stay active in your daily routine also plays a big role. Food should be consumed not by sitting in front of the TV or in a rush but in a relaxed manner and with leisure, paying attention to what you are eating. Enjoying the food with friends and family is also a part of the diet.

Drinking Too Much Wine Can Be Beneficial Because Drinking One Glass Is Deemed Beneficial

More isn't necessarily beneficial when it comes to consuming wine as part of the diet. Wine is allowed in moderate amounts, and a glass may have certain health benefits but drinking too much can have the opposite effect.

You Will Lose Weight Just By Following the Diet

Weight loss and good cardiovascular health are part of the diet but not just by following the diet but including exercise and physical activity throughout the day as well. People living on the Greek islands have an active lifestyle, and physical labor plays a major role in their maintaining good health.

Chapter3: Benefits of the Diet

It is not the diet itself that is beneficial, but the foods included in the diet that help affect the health positively. The nutrients and phytonutrients present in the foods, herbs, seasonings and fruits that are part of the Mediterranean diet are responsible for the benefits of the health. These benefits range from antiviral, antioxidant, antithrombic, anti-inflammatory and vasodilatory effects. So essentially when thinking about the benefits of the Mediterranean diet you should not think what it does for your health but rather what's inside the foods you are consuming that will trigger the health benefits.

The diet that we consume has six essential nutrients to keep us healthy and allow our body to function normally and effectively. These include carbohydrates, water, vitamins, minerals, fat, and proteins. Deficiency or imbalance of any of these nutrients can cause negative effects on the health. The ideal health and weight of a person is dependent on the sufficiency and balance of these nutrients. What the Mediterranean diet helps to do is maintain all these nutrients in a healthy amount through the intake of foods and high amount of vitamin, mineral, fiber and fatty acids. As it eliminates the intake of processed, junk and high-fat foods it allows to control the intake of health-harming fats and nutrients that contribute to the blockage of arteries, risk of developing heart diseases, obesity and overall ill health.

Apart from the nutrients that our body is supplied it is also supplied with phytochemicals which are beneficial to help fight diseases. Although these aren't as essential because not including them in our diet does not cause them to become deficient. Plant-based foods are abundant in phytonutrients and protects the plants from bugs, fungi, and germs. Currently, there are over 25000 phytonutrients while more are yet to be discovered. So having a diet rich in plant based foods ensure that you are adding a steady supply of phytonutrients to your diet. Following are some benefits of the Mediterranean diet as derived from different food sources:

Mediterranean Diet Food Sources

Fish

The two essential fatty acids that make up our diet are omega 3 and omega 6 which were in balance unless our food consumption choices disturbed that balance. Over time, the amount of omega 6 fatty acids increased up to 20 times more while that of omega 3 decreased. Omega 3 fatty acids are known to help prevent cardiovascular disease, arthritis, hypertension, obesity, and cancer and insulin resistance. Consuming fish on the Mediterranean diet helps include this essential fatty acid as it's a rich source.

Olive oil and olives

Olive oil and olives contain phenolic antioxidants that are found to protect against Alzheimer's disease, spinal cord injury, cerebral ischemia, Parkinson's disease, multiple sclerosis and peripheral neuropathy. The highest content of this phytonutrient is found in extra virgin olive oil and black olives, but these need to be consumed in moderation in order to keep the caloric intake under control.

Legumes

Another central food on this diet are legumes which include peas, soybeans, chickpeas, lentils, green beans, peanuts, alfalfa, clover, and dry beans. All these are also a rich source of phytonutrients that help prevent different diseases and disorders such as diabetes, coronary heart disease, inflammation, and high blood pressure.

Garlic

You can add different herbs and spices to flavor your food on the Mediterranean diet and a Garlic is a herb that isn't only good in taste but contains an essential phytonutrient allicin that has anticancer properties and contributes towards lowering the risk of cardiovascular disease.

Capers

Capers are a type of shrub that is frequently used in preparing many different cuisines and dishes on the Mediterranean diet such as chicken piccata, and eggplant caponata. It has numerous health benefits. It contains anti-diabetic, anti-atherosclerosis, antiviral, antioxidative, antimicrobial and immunomodulatory properties.

Additionally ponder over some of the following health benefits of the diet which have also been previously shown as validated by research studies:

Health Benefits of Mediterranean Diet

It helps prevent type 2 diabetes: This diet helps slow down digestion, is rich in fibers and help prevent spikes in blood sugar level all which contribute to preventing type 3 diabetes.

It helps prevent strokes and heart disease: Prime reasons for stroke and heart disease include consuming red meat, processed foods hard liquor and refined bread which are all discouraged in a Mediterranean diet.

It helps reduce Alzheimer's risk: Researchers validate the fact that this diet helps control blood vessel health, improve cholesterol and blood sugar levels which helps in reducing the risk of dementia and Alzheimer's.

It helps reduce the risk of Parkinson's: the Mediterranean diet is rich in antioxidants that prevent the cells from undergoing the damaging process known as oxidative stress, helping cut the risk of Parkinson's disease in half.

It helps keep agile: The nutrients that are included in the Mediterranean food diet plan can help reduce muscle weakness and other frailty signs by as much as 70 percent.

Chapter4: Concerns Associated With Mediterranean Diet

Like any other diet, there are some concerns voiced about the Mediterranean diet as well. There seems to be no doubt about the fact that a Mediterranean diet is good for the heart and helps reduce negative heart effects, but there are claims that it leads to obesity and weight gain. Obesity, as we know, is not good for the heart. Several studies in the European Union indicated that those who followed the Mediterranean diet became obese or overweight. However, that claim seems to be too farfetched to be true.

In order to validate that the Mediterranean diet itself does not cause obesity or heart disease a study was published in the American Journal of Clinical Nutrition which followed 23,597 male and female volunteers who were between age 20 and 86. The participants were part of a larger EU study that was investigating cancer and nutrition, however, for this particular study each participant's weight and height was measured to calculate their Body Mass Index. Participants were inquired in detail about their dietary pattern over the year which led the researchers to assign their Mediterranean diet adherence on a scale of 0 to 9.other variables that were accounted for each participant included their average caloric intake, physical activity, level of education and whether or not they smoke.

The study revealed that with the increase in age and caloric intake and if the participants smoked their BMI increased whereas as their physical activity and education level increased their BMI decreased. This led to proof that a high level of adherence to the Mediterranean diet, in fact, did not lead to an increase in BMI as was stipulated. Even when the researchers took the caloric intake out of the equation, they found that a higher adherence to the diet only led to a 0.21 increase in BMI in men and 0.05 increase in BMI in women.

If the Greeks were gaining weight and becoming obese in spite of following the foods recommended on the Mediterranean diet then it wasn't because of the foods, it was the likely result of other variables such as not being physically active and overeating.

Other concerns on the Mediterranean diet are the higher consumption of olive oil that people might partake without making other adjustments to their diet and lifestyle. This could lead to higher caloric intake and doing the opposite of what it's supposed to do. It is important when following the Mediterranean diet to keep the calories in check as well. The reason that the Mediterranean diet has gained significance and popularity is due to the fact that at the time it was discovered the people living in the Mediterranean countries had very low in fact no risk of heart diseases and death did not occur as a cause of cardiovascular risk. At that time, the American food culture had started to sway away from a healthy diet, and their consumption of junk foods started appearing in the form of different heart diseases.

Another thing to note on the diet is that adopting only part of it will not work or work positively. Eating healthy vegetables on the one hand but consuming cheeseburgers on the other in the name of cheat days will have no effect on health because any positive effect that is being generated will simultaneously be cancelled out by the consumption of high-fat foods. So you can't argue that you're eating vegetables and healthy fruits but still see no change in your health when, in fact, you are indulging in other fast foods as well. In order to benefit from the Mediterranean diet, it is very important to adopt its diet plan as suggested and stick to it, avoiding any other kinds of foods that impede its progress.

While alcohol is part of the diet in moderation, it might not suit everyone as it has its own health risks and concerns, in the long run, consuming a glass of wine each day might not be very beneficial for health, and if you are an avid wine drinker, it might be difficult for you to limit even your wine consumption to the recommended dose allowed each day on the diet.

Chapter5: The Research

Myths regarding the Mediterranean diet have largely been debunked I'd say, and strong evidence has been pouring in favor of the Mediterranean diet. Researchers conclude that it can help reduce heart risk, and there is strong evidence for that. One interesting and recent research study that tracked participants for ten years concludes that the Mediterranean diet is good for all types of people. Whether you want to lose weight, start living a healthier life, decrease your risk of developing cardiovascular diseases and other related health problems, the Mediterranean diet provides a well-rounded solution to achieve all your health goals.

According to the researchers at The Harokopio University, the diet is a beneficial intervention for people of all age groups in both genders, and its health implications aren't limited to those with heart diseases. It benefits even healthy people. The research participants of this study were 2,500 Greek adults between the ages of 18 and 89 whose dietary habits were monitored for a period of ten years. Data gathered at the end of the study was compared with data gathered at the start of the study and five years into the research, which took an in-depth look at the participants' lifestyle, diet, and medical records. The closer the person follows the Mediterranean diet the lower their chances are of developing heart diseases, it was found. Furthermore, what's interesting is the finding that even following 11 out of 55 options listed in the study, the participants were able to decrease their risk of developing a heart disease by 47 percent.

It's important to note here that this diet that I set out to research is not some fad diet. A number of researchers and cardiologists all agree that it might just be the key to unlocking your weight loss and healthy eating, and scientific research backs it. Of all the diets that people follow the Mediterranean diet is one of the few recommended by doctors as a way to develop a healthy lifestyle and system which is easy to follow.

I believe that if it was the Greeks natural way of having food the Americans can adopt the same model, but one problem that could be faced was our dependence on the quick and dirty fast foods. We live in a hyper-busy world where everyone feels that they are running out of time. Our work hours are longer, there is more pressure in life to do all the things that we want to do and accomplish and certainly there is a lot less focus on our health and what we are eating, let alone feeding our kids.

When you come to think about it, it's not that difficult to follow the Mediterranean lifestyle, and it certainly shouldn't be, and that is what my research aims to found it. The study is based on two hypotheses:

- First , whether the Mediterranean diet helps develop a healthier lifestyle
- Second, whether it is easy to retain this lifestyle

It's important to look at this diet from these two perspectives because we as Americans are increasingly drifting away from a healthy lifestyle. It is not only our food consumption that is unhealthy but a whole set of activities that are contributing to our unhealthy lifestyle. The one problem that I see evident in today's teenagers is the need to stay connected. Smartphones have become the lifeblood for this generation; it is troubling to see the young, and the old both focus more on their social followers and the likes and less on their diets. The fact that, today, we prefer to have our food while glued to one digital screen or the other, is even more worrisome because this behavior is a significant cause of obesity. A report in the American Journal of Clinical Nutrition looks at how attention to what we are eating affects our food intake, and no doubt, it has serious consequences. Distracted or hurried eating can result in you eating more, and we all know where overeating leads to. Researchers found out that if you're eating while you are distracted, the "I am full" signal that the brain has to send is delayed because you are not mindful of what you're eating, and thus that information isn't processed. There is no memory registered in your brain that you have eaten, and this could lead to as much as a 25 percent increase in food intake than what you are supposed to have.

Other evident unhealthy habits that we are all guilty of include endless hours of gaming and computing, and of course, sleeping late. The overuse of technology is interfering with our healthy sleeping habits, and nevertheless that is also part of maintaining a healthy lifestyle.

The reason that I am emphasizing on a holistic and healthy lifestyle is because that's how the Mediterranean diet benefits people who follow it. The rules of the diet are quite simple, but what makes a difference is whether along with eating healthy foods that are recommended you are adopting other healthy habits as well. The benefits of adopting a healthy routine and lifestyle go a long way in preventing diseases and help achieve overall good health. A few benefits of adopting a healthy diet routine are mentioned below:

Benefits of a healthy diet routine:

It enhances feelings of happiness

Healthy eating not only benefits people by helping them get rid of excess fat, but it helps them feel better about themselves. A research study that looked at 300 young adults in New Zealand found that the higher fruits and vegetable intake recommended to them resulted in them feeling calmer and more energized leading to overall happiness and better mood. The results were observed for only the day the food was consumed but lingered on until the next day.

It adds freshness to the skin

A study conducted by scientists at the University of Nottingham found out that those who ate more fresh produce had more attractive photographs than people with a suntan. In another study, participants who included more vegetables and fruits in their diet appeared more attractive than those with lower intake of fruits and vegetables. What you eat affects the body and the system from the inside, and when you eat healthy, it eventually shows up on your skin.

It helps enhance workout performance

A healthy diet and healthy foods are without a doubt the essential to enhancing your muscles, improving endurance or boosting recovery. A research study published in the Journal of Applied Physiology concluded that participants who drank 16 ounces of organic beetroot juices every day for six days increased their cycling by 16% compared to the placebo group.

It helps improve brain function

Eating healthy such as following a Mediterranean diet can also lead to improved brain function. A research from the National Institutes found that people following this diet lifestyle were less prone to develop brain infarcts that are small regions of dead tissue that can cause cognitive problems in a person.

Consuming unhealthy foods puts a person at a 66 percent increased risk of productivity loss. Consuming junk foods or those with too much spice or oil can lead you to feel bloated and prevents you from performing optimally.

The Mediterranean diet is not just about eating the recommended foods but also about adopting and following healthy habits that protect our body and heart.

This research is part of a three series research that looks on different diets and their effectiveness. The Mediterranean diet is a wholesome approach to healthy eating inspired from the Greek dietary lifestyle and my curiosity to find out how effective it really is for people of all ages, led me to it. This research looks at the two perspectives of adopting this diet helping people understand how they can live a healthier and risk-free life by making small changes to their diet and how it can be sustained over time, meaning adopted as a lifestyle change that is there to stay

Participants

For the purpose of this research, 5 participants were chosen. All of them consented to voluntarily participation. The participants chosen were between the ages of 18-45. Three male and two female participants were selected at different life stages. One male and female participant were obese with certain heart risks while two other participants were obese. The remaining male participant was healthy. The health variance in participants is chosen to validate the findings of the adoption of the Mediterranean diet for both genders and across different ages as well as for healthy, obese, and at-heart-risk people.

Study

This research study took place for a period of six months in which participants were given a complete health and food plan to follow. They were advised to join the gym or do other exercises as suitable to them. The participants had to follow the given diet plan which was developed after much research and keeping in mind the caloric intake for each participant. Participants were advised to adopt other healthy habits as well such as developing a set sleeping routine, limiting the use of technology, limiting sugar, and junk intake. The participants gathered for a meet up each week to take down their results, progress and discuss any difficulties that they were facing in following the diet plan. Below is a sample diet plan that the participants were given to follow:

	Day1	Day2	Day3	Day4	Day5	Day6	Day7
Breakfast	pancakes	Yogurt granola parfait	Chive and Goat Cheese Frittata	Pancakes and fresh raspberries	Creamy and crunchy yogurt	Peanut butter bagel and chocolate milk	Pita with ricotta spread and raisins
Lunch	Chickpea salad	Vegetable pot pie	Turkey and Artichoke Sandwich	Mediterranean grilled sea bass	Vegetarian pita sandwich with Greek cucumber yogurt sauce	Pizza with salad	Souvlaki Lamb and Rice
Snack	Crackers and dip	Chickpea salad	Chickpea spread	Vegetables and sweet sour cream dip	Crackers with sweet, creamy spread	Pineapple smoothie	Smoothie
dinner	Chicken kabobs	Tomato and mozzarella sandwich	Mediterranean grilled sea bass	Frittata and baklava	Mediterranean sweet and sour chicken	Souvlaki Lamb and Rice	Basil shrimp summer salad

	Day1	Day2	Day3	Day4	Day5	Day6	Day7
Calories	1469	1548	1543	1532	1579	1561	1574
Fat	25g	41g	50g	56g	36g	51g	39g
Carbs	209g	246g	169g	153g	226g	215g	228g
protein	81g	58g	110g	98g	80g	62g	86g

Note: each participant was compensated for the foods listed on the diet plan

Results:

Results for all the participants showed positive effects. Each of them reported feeling lighter and more motivated to continue the diet. However, participants agreed that the Mediterranean diet wasn't as difficult as following other kinds of diet plans because it requires making subtle shifts to dietary pattern to be able to consume healthier foods. Lab test results from participants who suffered from the risk of heart disease revealed after 6 months that they were able to lower their risk of developing cardiovascular disease but in this short period of time the change which came forth was minimal. Nevertheless, it was a positive finding.

	Participant1	Participant2	Participant3	Participant4	Participant5
Weight before the diet	318	296	290	321	187
Weight after the diet	237	221	186	226	164
Total weight loss	81	75	104	95	23

Cholesterol	Participant1	Participant2
Cholesterol level before the diet	369	342
Cholesterol level after the diet	211	224

(Total Cholesterol)

Findings and Conclusion:

Whether you are slim or fat, the fact is that you should be at a healthy weight according to your height and BMI. When we talk about being slim, we often forget the aspect of weight loss that not everyone can achieve an unrealistic weight. Your weight must be according to your physique. This misconception of having a certain weight that makes you slim causes many people to follow fad diets and destroy their health in the process. If you're not healthy then mind you, you are not slim either. Being slim means, you are healthy to enjoy life's bounty.

Bending too much on one side of the coin causes problems for many people, and that is what happens when people follow unrealistic diets that are not based on any scientific proof. The fact is that the Mediterranean diet comes with a proof of an entire generation that has been found to live healthy lives well into older ages, and subsequent researches have validated the claims made by this popular diet.

My research participants who were strictly on the above-mentioned diet plan with some variations here and there in their meals managed to follow it easily. However, two participants reported some amount of difficulty because they weren't used to eating any fruits or vegetables. Most of the people I assume are fond of fruits and vegetables, and those are the very things that make up the majority of the diet plan in a Mediterranean diet. The other three participants had lesser problems following the menu plan because they were already used to including fruits and vegetables to their diet and were health conscious as well.

A major difficulty across participants that was revealed was the adoption of an exercise or gym plan in their routine to keep them healthy. No participant was previously used to exercising or even walk or running. This is a problem faced by a majority of people that can't seem to take time out for exercise. All participants reported that including the said foods in their diet wasn't as difficult as taking time out for exercise. However, they started by including a 5-minute walk and them moving onto other routines that suit their schedule in the six months period.

In today's world, where everyone seems to be running after something, and there doesn't seem to be any time for the important things, such as taking care of your health, almost everyone uses this as an excuse for not exercising. People who follow the Mediterranean diet and even the research participants revealed that even short period of exercise whether it was running, yoga or a mere walk around the corner helped them feel better and lighter. A light walk after dinner helps get fresh air and helps digest the food faster.

Almost all participants lost weight while on the Mediterranean diet plan. The two participants who had developed a risk of heart diseases were also found to have lowered their risk because of including healthier foods in their diet. Although in the short period of 6 months, this decrease was somewhat minor but it was evidently there. However, the focus of my research was majorly on their weight loss and the adoption difficulty of the diet and on both fronts, I saw the participants achieving positive results. Adopting a healthy diet isn't difficult but what matters most is making those changes to your diet that stick with you. In the beginning, participants found it difficult to stick to only vegetables and fruits. The mere thought that they could no longer consume a burger or a hotdog was daunting as the first few weeks progressed, and they started to see positive changes it became apparent that it was for their own good.

Participants also reported feeling good about themselves overall as the research progressed. Gradually they started becoming used to the new lifestyle that included eating healthy meals, setting a time schedule, and including some amount and form of exercise in their daily schedule. As you are not limiting your diet or caloric intake on this diet, participants did not experience any of the typical diet symptoms such as headaches, starvation, low blood pressure, tiredness, or lethargy. Instead, your caloric intake remains more or less the same except that it now comes from healthy sources instead of consuming fats or sugars. This suggests that there are absolutely no drawbacks or side effects of the diet and merely what you are doing is shifting from a non-healthy lifestyle to a healthier one. However, the shift could be slow and bother you to the extent that you may not be able to consume your favorite high-fat foods any longer. Other than that, I believe every person has the power to follow the Mediterranean diet if they want to live a healthy and active life and lower their chances of developing cardiovascular risks later on in life.

Chapter6: How to Achieve Success on the Mediterranean Diet

So now that you have seen the results and findings of my research study that have largely been positive I will talk about YOUR success and how YOU can achieve the same positive changes in your life, helping you to lead a healthier life. For most people giving up their favorite junk foods is difficult but I believe it's not as hard as we assume it is.

We are just used to that greasy taste and just as easily, we became used to it in a matter of some days we can undo it and adopt other tastes that are appealing to our tastes buds. It just a matter of choosing the right flavors and seasonings in our food to create the taste that we were previously used to. That is what I advised my research participants as well those were finding it difficult to eat the vegetables. Vegetables have also endured the blame of being boring and tasteless, but you don't need to continue taking them like it.

You can make your veggies interesting, colorful, and tasty by adding spices and seasonings. That the best part of the Mediterranean diet that it doesn't limit a lot of foods for you. It allows you to consume whatever you like with the only condition that it should be healthy. The majority of your caloric intake should be from vegetables, fruits, and you will soon see that very little calories are left to be consumed from other sources and those will definitely not be the unhealthy ones. The only thing you should eliminate from your diet is sugar and limit your intake of dairy products.

Here are my personal tips for making the Mediterranean diet easy for you to follow, based on observations of my research participants:

10 Easy to Follow Tips to Success

Buy your ingredients in bulk

Once you know or have a meal to follow instead of running out each day to find your ingredients to prepare the meals of the day go through the plan once and do your grocery shopping for the week on one day. This will save you time and effort, helping you avoid the panic last minute. Olive oil is the main ingredient to cook your dishes in and can be expensive than regular oil. You can purchase a large bottle and use it cautiously.

Plan and prepare ahead

Once you buy our ingredients in bulk, you should also prepare, plan and stock your foods in advance so that it saves you any trouble of getting late to work and feeling like your diet is restricting you. If you put all things into perspective, you can really make it happening for you but it will take some getting used to.

If eating out, choose Greek cuisine

Eating out can be unavoidable at times and when you do you don't want to appear like a snob who's above the rest especially when you are out with your friends. Friends don't necessarily understand that you are dieting or trying to adopt a healthy lifestyle and almost always they will try to push you off track. You can avoid such a situation by carefully choosing a Greek dish or stick to a gorgeous and fulfilling salad. No one will doubt your eating habits. Just remember the foods you have to avoid and make sure you avoid them.

As much as you can, consume fresh foods

Your kitchen will undergo some changes when you switch to a Mediterranean diet, and I can most definitely tell you that you will be saving some money as well along the way as you make the changes. All the expensively packaged ready to cook foods and fast foods you were used to consuming will now have to be cut down and replaced with veggies and fruits and these you must try to consume as much fresh and organic as you can.

Include some tasteful herbs

Eating healthy doesn't mean you have to eat boring and if you can add some herbs and spices to make your food taste good, then you must. Store some spices such as allspice, oregano, cilantro, mint, parsley, basil, and garlic in your kitchen and use them when cooking your foods. Again try to use fresh spices because dry spices can be potent but if you use them minimally, you can go ahead with it.

Roast your veggies

You can also save time in preparing your meals by cutting a batch of veggies for the week and roasting them for 15-20 minutes. You can use this bath of veggies to add to your dishes, seasons the pasta or even eat cold.

These are some of the general tips that will help you prepare yourself for the Mediterranean diet easily and seriously. When you become well organized, you will realize that it is, in fact, easy to follow it as it does not come with a lot of restrictions or do's and don'ts. Your food choices are very clear and straightforward, and you have to make overall life changes to achieve your goals however, this isn't to say you should change overnight, but you can at least start one day and aim to achieve the healthy routine in a time frame of 2-3 weeks. That is the latest when the last research participant told me that he was now completely following the diet plan and exercising as well. I am assuming it should not take you more time than that to make the switch.

Here are additional tips to help you remember your food choices:

Swap your butter and margarine with olive oil

By now you must be clear that you have to cook your foods in olive oil but it also implies that if you were cooking your foods using butter or margarine or having them for breakfast, you have to put a limit to it. Olive oil is recommended on the Mediterranean diet as a core component to cooking dishes in because it is a rich source of monounsaturated fats that are good for the heart. If you find the extra virgin oil too expensive you can use it limitedly when cooking and use other healthy oil substitutes such as canola or walnut oil which are also rich in monounsaturated fats and omega 3 fatty acids.

Alter your protein intake

On this diet, you should be getting the majority of your protein from chicken, turkey, beans, fish, nuts, and other plants. Red meat should be off limits which will also lower your intake of saturated fats. If you find these changes hard to make, make them little by little. Add fish to the menu twice a week, salmon and tuna are god choices in this regard to start with as these are a rich source of omega 3 fatty acids which contribute towards good heart health. It is okay to indulge your meat cravings once a while, and you can do that by adding diced meat to your pasta or choosing the lean cut and limiting your portion size to only 3-4 ounces.

Stock up on vegetables

No one likes eating vegetables, but the basis of the Mediterranean diet lies in making friends with your greens. You should be getting a lot of those in your meals. Include 3-8 servings of vegetables each day which

Is anywhere between ½ a cup to 2 cups. You can decide your vegetables yourself as they give you a variety of antioxidants and vitamins to pile up on. You can prepare a vegetable soup or have them roasted; really, there are unlimited ways of making your vegetables interesting to have when you want to have it.

Include whole grains to your diet

You can lavishly add whole grain foods to your diet but make sure they aren't the "refined" form of grains you are eating. For example, you can include quinoa as a side dish with your meals, which just takes 20 minutes to cook. Barley is also a good option as it is filling and full of fiber. Oatmeal can be a good choice for breakfast. Make sure any whole grain that you buy has "whole" or "whole grain" written on the package.

Chapter 7: 15 Delicious Recipes

Following the Mediterranean diet isn't particularly difficult and all you need to do is remember the foods that have to be included in your diet while steering clear of those which you have to avoid. Compared with other diets, I find the Mediterranean diet easy to follow as there is no particular calorie count from fats, proteins, or carbohydrates to keep track of. This essentially leaves a lot of room for having healthy foods to your liking in a day as your diet intake isn't limited.

However, as the Mediterranean diet suggests that you should increase the intake of fruits and vegetables in your diet along with whole grains, you need to have different dishes at the ready to consume because you can't be eating raw veggies and fruits every day. For that matter, having a diet plan and recipes to follow comes in handy especially when you are in a time crunch. You can follow the diet plan given in this book for participants and as you learn more about the diet, make personal adjustments to suit yourself. The recipes for the dishes listed in the diet plan are given below:

Pancakes:

Serves: 5

Ingredients:

- Low-fat yogurt: 1 ½ cup
- Egg: 1 large
- Whole wheat pancake mix: 1
- Fat-free milk: ¾ cup

Preparation Method:

1. In a bowl, combine the yogurt, pancake mix, and milk.
2. Serve with a cup of strawberries

Note: since the recipe serves five people, you can store away the remaining four servings for later if there is no one else having it with you.

Chickpea Salad

Ingredients:

- Canned chickpeas: ½ of a 15-ounce can
- Olive oil: 2 tsp
- Chopped white onion: ¼ cup
- Chopped green pepper: ¼ cup
- Sliced black olives: 1 tbsp
- Ground black pepper: ¼ tsp
- White vinegar: 1 ½ tbsp

Preparation Method:

1. Combine and mix all the ingredients thoroughly in a bowl
2. Serve with 2 cups of romaine lettuce

Chicken Kabobs

Ingredients:

- Raw chicken breast: 4 ounces
- Fat-free Italian Dressing: ¼ cup
- Chopped white onion: ¼ cup
- Chopped green pepper: ¼ cup
- Grape tomatoes: 10

Preparation Method:

1. Slice the chicken breast into chunks and marinate overnight for 30 minutes
2. Slice the green pepper and white onion into chunks as well.
3. Alternate the chicken, pepper, onion, and tomatoes on skewers and grill
4. Serve with pita bread if you like

Yogurt Granola Parfait

Ingredients:

- light fruit-flavored yogurt: 6 ounces
- Raspberries: 1 cup
- Low-fat granola: 2 tbsp

Preparation Method:

1. Layer one-third of the yogurt, raspberries and granola in a wide mouth glass and continue until the quantities are used.
2. Enjoy fresh

Vegetable Pot Pie

- Vegetable pot pie: 1 (preferably Amy's)

Preparation Method:

1. Follow the instructions on packet to prepare the pie
2. Serve with grape tomatoes

Chickpea Spread

Serves: 2

Ingredients:

- Chickpeas: ½ an ounce of can
- Olive oil: 2 tsp
- Minced Garlic: 1 clove
- Lemon juice: 1 tbsp
- Salt: ¼ tsp
- Ground cumin: ¼ tsp

Preparation Method:

1. Mash chickpeas in a bowl and add all the remaining ingredients
2. Mix well
3. Serve with a cup of broccoli flowerets

Tomato and Mozzarella Sandwich

- 6-inch French baguette roll: 1
- Mozzarella cheese (shredded): 1/3 cup
- Red tomatoes (large): 2
- Dried basil: as desired
- Dried oregano: as desired

Preparation Method:

1. Slice the baguette roll in half, lengthwise, sprinkle with cheese and bake it for 4-6 minutes in the toaster at 250 degrees.
2. Take it out when cheese begins to melt and sprinkle with basil and oregano as desired.
3. Cut the tomatoes in half and layer them over the cheese.
4. Serve fresh.

Turkey and Artichoke Sandwich

Ingredients

- Whole wheat bread: 2 slices
- Light mayonnaise: 1 tbsp

- Artichoke hearts: 4-6
- Reduced fat mozzarella cheese: 1/3 cup (shredded)
- Sliced turkey breast: 3 ounces

Preparation Method:

1. Apply mayonnaise to the whole wheat bread slices.
2. Add artichoke hearts, cheese, and sliced turkey breast.
3. Serve with a cup of red grapes or 15 baby carrots

Mediterranean Grilled Sea Bass

Serves: 4

Ingredients:

- Lemons: 2
- Olive oil: 3 tbsp
- Fresh oregano leaves (chopped): 1 tbsp
- Ground coriander: 1 tsp
- Salt: 1¼ tsp
- Whole sea bass: 2
- Ground black pepper: 1/4 tsp
- Oregano sprigs: 2 large

Preparation Method:

1. Preheat gas grill at medium heat or prepare charcoal fire
2. Grate 1 tbsp of lemon peel from one lemon and squeeze lemon juice worth 2 tbsp. Cut lemon slices and wedges from the remaining lemon halves.
3. Mix lemon juice and peel, coriander, salt and chopped oregano
4. Rinse the fish and when dry, make three slashes on both sides.
5. Sprinkle the fish with pepper and salt, inside out and insert lemon slices inside fish cavities

6. Put it in a baking dish and rub with oil. Let it stand for 15 minutes at room temperature
7. Grease the grill rack light and place fish. Cook it for 12-14 minutes; test it with a fork and flip.
8. Cut the fish along the backbone from head to tail. Pull out the rib bones and backbone and discard.
9. Transfer fish to a platter and serve with lemon wedges.

Mediterranean Sweet and Sour Chicken

Ingredients:

- Olive oil: 2 tsp
- Salt: ¼ tsp
- Skinless chicken thighs: 8 (small)
- Garlic clove: 2
- Chicken broth: ½ cup
- Real wine vinegar: ¼ cup
- Cornstarch: 2 tsp
- Brown Sugar: 2 tsp
- Salad olives: ¼ cup
- Mission figs: ¾ cup
- Baby arugula: 1 bag

Preparation Method:

1. Heat oil over medium-high heat until very hot in a non-stick skillet. Sprinkle chicken with salt and cook for 20 minutes or until it is brown and take out on plate
2. Stir the garlic on skillet for 30 seconds
3. Mix the broth, cornstarch, sugar, and vinegar in a cup with wire whisk.
4. Add the broth mixture to the skillet and bring to boil. Cook it until the sauce thickens. Stir in the onions and figs.

5. Serve hot with arugula.

Chive and Goat Cheese Frittata

Serves: 4

Ingredients:

- Eggs: 8 (large)
- Milk: ½ cup
- Salt: ½ tsp
- Ground black pepper: 1/8 tsp
- Tomato: 1 (medium)
- Chopped fresh chives: 2 tbsp
- Margarine: 2 tsp
- Goat cheese: 1.2 a package

Preparation Method:

1. Preheat oven to 375 degrees
2. Mix eggs, milk, salt, and pepper in a medium bowl with fork and add diced tomato and chopped chives
3. In a non-stick pan melt the margarine over medium heat and add egg and goat cheese. Cook for 4 minutes until the frittata begins to set.
4. Place skillet in oven and bake for 10 minutes. Check by inserting knife in the center. It should come out clean.
5. Serve hot.

Basil Shrimp Summer Salad

Ingredients:

- Shrimps: 9 large size or 12 medium size
- White wine vinegar: ¼ cup
- Olive oil: 1 tsp

- Chopped fresh basil: 1/8 cup
- Dried basil: 1 tsp
- Romaine lettuce: 2 cups

Preparation Method:

1. Prepare basil marinade by mixing white wine vinegar, olive oil, lemon juice, fresh and dried basil
2. Marinate the shrimps with basil marinade for 30 minutes or overnight.
3. Grill until cook and add romaine lettuce for added flavor on top
4. Serve with a cup of blueberries

Additional Recipes

Mediterranean Pasta Salad

Serves: 4

Ingredients:

- Multigrain farfalle: 8 ounce
- Lemon juice: 1 lemon
- Olive oil: 2 tsp
- Artichoke can: 1 (13.5 ounces)
- Chopped Mozzarella cheese: 8 ounces
- Chopped bottled roasted red bell pepper: ¼ cup
- Fresh parsley: ¼ cup (chopped)
- Frozen peas: ½ cup

Preparation Method:

1. Cook pasta omitting salt and fat

2. Meanwhile combine lemon juice and olive oil in a large bowl and stir well. add cheese, bell pepper, parsley, and artichoke hearts and combine well.
3. Add the pasta to peas and artichoke mixture and mix well to combine
4. Serve warm.

Calories per serving: 420, Fat per serving: 20g, Protein per serving: 20g, Carbohydrates per serving: 50g

Mediterranean Tuna

Serves: 6

Ingredients:

- Tuna (drained and flaked): 2 cans
- Mayonnaise dressing with olive oil: ¼ cup
- Chopped pitted olives: ¼ cup
- Roasted red peppers: ¼ cups
- Sliced green onions: 2
- Small capers: 1 tbsp
- Whole wheat bread: 6 slices

Preparation Method:

1. Combine all ingredients in a bowl except bread and toss well
2. Serve with bread and greens

Calories per serving: 190, Fat per serving: 6g, Protein per serving: 18g, Carbohydrate per serving: 13 g

Stuffed Tomatoes

Serves: 4

Ingredients:

- Tomatoes: 2 large
- Packaged garlic croutons: ½ cup
- Crumbled goat cheese: ¼ cup
- Pitted kalamata olives (sliced): ¼ cup
- Reduced fat vinaigrette: 2 tbsp
- Chopped fresh thyme: 2 tbsp

Preparation Method:

1. Preheat the boiler add cut tomatoes in half (crosswise)
2. Empty and discard the seeds. Cut out the pulp and transfer to a bowl. It should leave you with two shells.
3. Add croutons, olives, dressing, thyme, and goat cheese to a pulp and mix well.
4. Insert the mixture into the hollowed tomatoes
5. Place them in the broiler pan until cheese minutes.
6. Serve fresh and hot.

Calories per serving: 103, Fat per serving: 7g. Carbohydrates per serving: 8g, Protein per serving: 3g

Chapter 8: Conclusion

The Mediterranean diet is essentially the diet of the common man. However, the distinction is between the common man of the Mediterranean countries and the western countries. In the west, the diet that is followed is far from healthy. People have strayed far away from eating healthy and nutritious foods and rely more on easy to cook, ready to eat meals as well as fast foods. This could be attributed to the busy life schedule of the people where every man is for and on his own. This kind of lifestyle inevitably gives rise to a culture that is in a rush and built upon quick foods, so as to say.

It is seen that the people of the West started encountering frequent weight problems as well as heart problems, all of which is largely the result of an unhealthy diet. In order to lose weight and switch to a healthier lifestyle, it became imperative to find a solution, and when researchers looked towards the diet and health patterns of people living in Greece and surrounding regions, they found that that the people there were comparatively healthier.

It is all in one's diet- what you are consuming day in and day out. If all the people were to become conscious of everything that they put in their mouths at all times of the day, they would realize how near or far they are from healthy eating. The fact is, we don't count the foods outside of our three meals as part of our diet, and therein lies the problem. If you're eating healthy three times a day but not otherwise because everyone has frequent food cravings, then you're on a quick path to weight gain and subsequent health problems.

In order to lose weight and keep yourself healthy, you have to be conscious and aware of what you are eating at all times and enjoy it. This was the fact most evident in the diet patterns of the people of the Mediterranean countries – that they share their food with friends and family over laughter, and their meals consist mostly of healthy vegetables and fruits. To satisfy their cravings they, don't resort to fast food or other junk food but consume whole wheat foods. Wine is also an essential part of the diet, but the intake is limited. All these things in the subsequent research pointed towards the fact that there indeed is a need to make changes to what you are eating and how you are eating it if you want to be healthy.

My diet came to the same results. The world over, the Mediterranean diet is regarded as the best and most effective diet for heart patients, and there is no doubt in that. Two of my research participants had increased cholesterol, and soon after switching to the diet, the condition became under control. Other participants lost weight, and the most amazing thing is that they all started to feel fresher and healthier overall since they started on the Mediterranean diet. The fact is when you are light and healthy; you don't feel lethargic or fatigued as usually is the case when you have consumed heavy food. That creates a big difference and contributes to a person's overall health and wellbeing in different ways.

When you are eating light and healthy, you tend to feel more alert and awake. Our bodies are running on a mechanism, and we need to take care of that mechanism. But that mechanism is delicate, and as soon as we start neglecting it, the consequences appear soon after. Just like a car needing regular maintenance and upgrades to keep it running in optimal condition, our bodies need the right diet to keep it working efficiently and effectively. As we get older or even in the young generation, we see that this norm of eating healthy food is lost. Due to our hectic routines, we tend to rely increasingly on ready to cook meals and fast foods, destroying our health. There is a dire need to start eating healthy in order to stay fit.

My research on this diet has led me to believe in comparison with other diets that the Mediterranean diet is easy to follow. There is necessarily no limit on the amount of calories, fat or protein that you have to intake which essentially makes everything very easy to follow. If you have read my previous book in which I have talked about the effectiveness of the ketogenic diet, you would understand the reference. Just as a short reference, I would add that the ketogenic diet requires participants to limit their fat intake and increase the protein and carb intake in order to kick start the keto process in the body.

We see that in this diet, there are no such requirements. So you are essentially free to eat anything without worrying about the calories. The only condition is that it should be healthy. There are only a very few limitation on the Mediterranean diet such as restricting having meat to once a month and restricting the amount of wine to a glass. Other than that, you will find that it is easy to follow, and so my research participants thought as well.

I would personally like to add here that any kind of diet is going to go in vain unless you are determined to make a change in your life. I remember a time when I was overweight, and although it was only by a few pounds, I understood how easily it could escalate and go into the obese range. Initially, I paid no attention to it until my friends started to tease me, and before I started taking it seriously, I had turned fat. I realized this when my jeans wouldn't fit me anymore. This was a major blow to me. I advise anyone who asks for diet recommendation to first make a commitment to yourself that you want to lose weight and live healthy. When you stand true to your commitment only, then you will start to see the changes from a diet because you would be working with them and not just following rules for them to happen.

In order to find your success on the diet, you can add exercise to your daily schedule as well. Whether it is a ten minutes walk, treadmill, gym or simple jumping jacks, start doing it. It was one of the other things evident in the lifestyle of the people of the Mediterranean countries that they were very active. This essentially makes a lot of difference and contributes to good health overall when you allow your body to move and keep your mechanism in running. All your muscles should get equal treatment and should remain in action in order for them to work well and remain efficient. My research participants included exercise as well and found out that it was helping them become active in life overall.

As an end note, start with making a mindset change to find your success with the Mediterranean diet and then commit to making a lifestyle change of eating healthy food. Once you start switching your unhealthy foods with healthy choices, pair your efforts with exercise for maximum benefit. Remember that change isn't easy, but it is very beneficial if you are accepting of it.

www.ingramcontent.com/pod-product-compliance
Lightning Source LLC
Chambersburg PA
CBHW071133280526
45787CB00003B/1267